HOW TO BUY CBD OIL

The Beginners Guide to CBD Hemp Oil

Discover the 5 Important Considerations Required Selecting the Best CBD Oil for Pain, Anxiety and Health

Learn How to Make CBD Oil

EMA HAWKINS

Copyright

All rights reserved. No part of this publication may be reproduced, distributed, or transmitted in any form or by any means, including photocopying, recording, or other electronic or mechanical methods, without the prior written permission of the publisher, except in the case of brief quotations embodied in critical reviews and certain other noncommercial uses permitted by copyright law. Copyright © by Ema Hawkins

CONTENTS

PART 1: A BEGINNER'S GUIDE TO CBD OIL

INTRODUCTION TO CBD

Cannabidiol, CBD for short, is one of more than 80 cannabinoids in the cannabis plant.

It is by no means a new discovery. But recent advancements in research, scientific studies, and acceptance by the general population have put CBD, and in fact CBD oil on the map.

However, the challenge is that people are confused about what CBD actually is and many people assume it is marijuana and that it can get you high, which is false.

Cannabidiol is a non psychoactive chemical produced by cannabis plants like cannabis and hemp.

Cannabis is a genus of flowering plant in the cannabis family with many species including hemp.

This means that both marijuana and hemp belong to the same group of plants marked by common characteristics.

Most of us are more familiar with the cannabis string called marijuana that has been bred specifically to produce high levels of THC, which is the principal psychoactive ingredient that gets you high.

CBD stands for cannabidiol. It is also a compound that is found in cannabis. If you look at cannabis, there are two major compounds; THC which is the part that gets you high, and CBD.

They both are on totally different extremes.

So if you want to get the psychoactive effects of cannabis, you are going to look for high THC but if you want the healthy aspect of cannabis, you are going to look for as much CBD as possible.

One of the interesting things you find in the plant kingdom is that they contain complements or antagonistic chemical compounds that give different effects.

For example in the tea plant, we have caffeine and l-theanine and these tend to have a counterbalancing effect. They both tend to improve focus. But one tends to increase anxiety and the other tends to decrease anxiety.

CBD and THC sort of have that antagonist property.

Some of the things we see that are of great interest in what cannabidiol can do is that it increases neurogenesis.

And right now neurogenesis is felt to be one of the factors that are responsible for depression.

When you have a fall-off in the production of new neurons in the hippocampus, oftentimes what you have is an onset of depression.

And if people are not making new neurons they may be indeed depressed. CBD also decreases the apoptosis of neurons, decreased neuronal damage and cell death.

So it does look like it is neuroprotective in terms of neurodegenerative disease.

CBD has the ability to activate both the CB1 and CB2 receptors.

Theoretically, when the CB1 and CB2 receptors are functioning at full capacity, better and efficient medical conditions occur in the brain, the central nervous system, and in cells associated with your immune system.

Extraction

There's a lot of confusion about CBD; what it is and where it comes from.

Many people assume that CBD oil contains only CBD, whereas due to the CO_2 extraction method, it contains other cannabinoids such as CBD, CBDa, CBC, CBN, CBG, plus terpenes and flavonoids to give the full Entourage Effect.

Even though CBD is extracted from industrial hemp, industrial hemp is not the only source.

CBD oil can be made from both industrial hemp and marijuana, as they are both the cannabis plant.

Lots of CBD oil is produced with the CO_2 extraction method.

CBD oil can be made using any extraction method but CO_2 extraction is the best, since it preserves the terpenes and flavonoids. However, it does require expensive laboratory equipment.

Charlotte's web

Charlotte was a little girl who started having seizures soon after birth. By age three, she was having up to 300 seizures a week despite medications.

Once medical marijuana was tried on her, the seizures were limited to two or three per month.

However, they discovered it was not the THC part of the plant that helped; it was the cannabidiol (CBD) the plant contained.

They also discovered that they could extract the CBD oil without including the THC, and that the hemp plant (part of the same plant species) contained healthy CBD oil without THC.

Charlotte is 10 now and the great news is that she's thriving.

The Buzz

It did not take long for CBD oil to become a buzz within the mainstream, but the confusion continued as most people thought CBD oil was the marijuana plant with THC.

One of the things about cannabidiol is that it has had this explosion of interest in the last number of years such that there are now up to about 300 publications per year now on CBD.

The publications are all awash with its numerous benefits ranging from epilepsy in the 70s, drug abuse, anxiety, psychosis, Huntington's, MS, Alzheimer's, Parkinson's, depression and ALS.

It is very difficult to stay current with this field because it is increasing geometrically.

And I think it's increasing geometrically because people are realizing that this has a profound pervasive effect in biological systems.

...and not only in terms of medical interventions such as pain...

...but also for psychiatric interventions, such as anxiety, psychosis and probably even trauma.

HEALTH BENEFITS: WHY YOU SHOULD TAKE CBD OIL

First of all, we're deficient in CBD. The last time that we got a cannabinoid was probably in Mom's milk.

And so from that point on we have receptors in our systems that are waiting for CBD and other cannabinoids to come in and fill them up.

Once you get these receptors filled up then your cells can have the right activity, and great things could happen to your health response.

For instance, when you have anxiety or stress, it indicates that those receptors are looking for a CBD to calm them.

CBD is used for an unending list of medical conditions; anti-inflammatory, pain relief, stress and anxiety, insomnia, muscle spasms, seizures, Parkinson's, Crohn's disease, PTSD, epilepsy, heart disease, autism, ADHD and so on.

Your doctor may recommend CBD oil as either a preventive medicine, or for the treatment of various autoimmune disorders, as well as other conditions such as arthritis, multiple sclerosis, blood pressure, blood sugar diabetes, gastrointestinal disorders, bipolar disorders, schizophrenia, and more.

CBD oil may also be able to remedy any severe pain and/or nausea you may experience after undergoing chemotherapy.

CBD also plays an important role in skeletal remodeling.

And as we get older, we see more people getting osteoporosis and osteopenia.

So it is an important function that CBD oil can play in that area.

It also helps prevent strokes because of its neuroprotective elements.

It augments stem cells. We have heard a lot of research about stem cells and the benefit of stem cells.

What are stem cells?

Those are cells which allow every type of cell to develop in your body, so it's kind of like the baby cell that differentiates into every other type of cell.

HEMP

Hemp, also called industrial hemp, just like marijuana, is a member of the family of cannabis sativa plants.

Hemp is a cannabis plant that is harvested commercially for its seeds and stalks, which are used to produce a number of products including food, nutritional supplements, medicine, body care products, paper, and textiles.

All the raw hemp materials are imported from other countries, which is unfortunate because hemp is a great rotation crop for farmers.

As it grows, it inhales atmospheric CO_2, rids the soil of its toxins, and helps to curb soil erosion.

Cultivating hemp also does not require pesticides, and very little water is needed, which makes it more environmentally and economically friendly than traditional crops.

Now for the big shocker, the cultivation of hemp (which contains little or no THC) without permit was declared illegal in the United States under the Controlled Substances Act passed in 1970 because it came from the same plant family as marijuana.

So, all hemp products like hemp seeds are imported from places like Canada because you can't grow it in the United States.

You can't get high off of hemp because of the low chemical makeup of THC. Whereas marijuana has very high amounts of THC-especially the marijuana that is specifically bred to get you high.

So both hemp plants and marijuana contain CBD but marijuana contains THC. It is therefore possible to avoid the THC by sticking with CBD oil that has been extracted from hemp.

The History of Hemp

What is it about hemp that's so controversial?

Why is it always in the news lately?

And is it only because it's tied to medical marijuana?

Can it be good?

I'll leave the legal discussion to the lawyers. What I'm interested in are potential health benefits.

Hemp has the reputation as being this evil weed. But the medicinal history of hemp is quite fascinating.

As far back as the 1930s, there were medicinal hemp tinctures in almost every pharmacy in the United States.

Washington, Jefferson, Lincoln and all the presidents actually grew hemp, at least according to anecdotes. So it was legal to grow everywhere. And they could use it as they wanted.

As a matter of fact, some farmers in the colony of Virginia were required to grow hemp being industrially useful as fiber and very good for making clothes, paper, biodegradable plastics and a lot of other different industrial uses.

Ford thought it was strong enough to make a car out of it and he did. In fact one of the first Model Ts was actually made from hemp and it ran on hemp fuel

Hemp is a much more efficient way to make paper. In one acre of hemp, you can do ten times the amount of paper than one acre of trees.

So Hearst wanted hemp outlawed because he owned thousands of acres of forest.

So hemp was demonized and thought of as evil weed.

They put out propaganda films to make people afraid of hemp when in reality, that's one small use of hemp; the recreational use, which we call marijuana.

Marijuana was a slang term that they developed to make people afraid of hemp. Others were 'oh heck', 'Mary Jane', and so on.

In the 1930s, tinctures (a medicine made of a drug with an alcohol solvent) were made because the medicinal uses of hemp are just numerous.

We can talk about the cancer effects of hemp as well as how it helps with inflammation being very anti-inflammatory.

It also helps with seizures; it's very effective with PTSD for the vets.

There are about a dozen different cancers that have been studied in depth with hemp; from brain cancer to prostate cancer to pancreatic cancer, uterine cancer, cervical cancer prostate cancer- it's just so amazing.

There are chemicals that are called cannabinoids in the hemp plant, including THC and CBD as you already know.

THC is short for tetrahydrocannabinol. It is the psychoactive compound in the cannabis plant that gets you high if you smoke it.

But there's other cannabinoids.

One is called CBD cannabidiol. And it's very useful medicinally with no psychoactive component.

You have to heat the THC to make it become psychoactive.

So if you eat the plant as a super green smoothie, you are not going to get high off of that because you didn't superheat it.

HEMP OR MARIJUANA?

Wikipedia describes cannabis as marijuana, that is able to get you high when consumed recreationally.

In addition to that, if you Google the images for cannabis, you get pictures of hippies, Bob Marley, Rastafarians and smoking joints.

The same is true when you Google hemp.

Wikipedia comes up first, and hemp is described as industrial hemp typically found in the northern hemisphere.

And that it is a variety of the cannabis sativa plant species that are grown for industrial uses to produce products such as clothing, rope, canvas, paper and even textiles.

So you can see that even Google has a certain definition of what cannabis is, and it's confusing.

We need to clear the confusion about when it is marijuana and when it is hemp.

Cannabis may come from the same plant, but the species are very different.

They are different in appearance, for example, marijuana is a bush, has very broad leaves, and a tight bud. Whereas hemp grows very tall, up to 20 feet, and has skinny leaves concentrated at the top.

They are not only different in their appearance but they're also very different chemically.

Marijuana has high THC, anywhere from 5 to 35% and low CBD, whereas hemp, which has low THC, also has to have 0.3% or less to be legal.

It has high CBD and other cannabinoids.

The differences between hemp and marijuana could be used of the analogy between oranges and lemons for instance.

They both come from the citrus family but they're entirely different.

CBD Oil: Hemp or Cannabis?

There's a lot of confusion in the marketplace right now with the difference between hemp-based CBD oil and cannabis-derived CBD oil, but you shouldn't be confused at all.

If you take a look at the hemp-based CBD oil molecule and the cannabis-based CBD oil molecule, they're exactly the same. However, the hemp is a non-psychoactive plant that has 0.3% THC or less.

When you use CBD oil that comes from the cannabis plant essentially, you're also getting a different percentage of THC as well as other components of the cannabis-based plant like the terpenes, as well as three to four hundred other chemicals that are in there that interact together to produce what's called the entourage effect.

For the hemp base, you just have the CBD from the hemp as well as THC, but less than 0.3%.

The entourage effect means that all of these things work together to create a bigger and better effect as a medicine.

That's what a lot of people experience. You need to try them yourself.

Some people take hemp-based CBD oil, others prefer CBD based on the cannabis plant, and can't even tell the difference between them.

Some people take them and claim to experience better effects by using the whole plant-based CBD oil from the cannabis plant versus just using the hemp.

The takeaway really is to try it and see how you react to it separately.

And one of the other big differences is that you can actually purchase hemp-derived CBD oils online.

So you don't need a medical marijuana recommendation.

But the problem with those is that you don't know where they're coming from.

They could be coming from China, which is where a lot of the industrial hemp comes from or Canada.

But there are no controls so you don't know exactly what you're purchasing.

HOW CBD OIL WORKS IN YOUR BODY

Now that we know the difference between CBD extracted from the hemp plant and CBD extracted from the marijuana plant, let's discuss how CBD oil works in our body and what all the excitement about.

Scientists are rapidly discovering more and more benefits of CBD.

The big selling point being touted is that it is plant-based, safe, non-addictive in non euphoric.

CBD is a vital cannabinoid with therapeutic properties for numerous disorders that are even yet to be completely identified.

What scientists are discovering is that it is an anti-inflammatory, anticonvulsant, antioxidant an anti-psychotic agent, in potential medicine for epilepsy, oxidative injury, anxiety, PTSD and schizophrenia to just name a few.

When someone takes CBD, the compound goes into the endocannabinoid system, also called ECS, which is made up of receptors throughout our body and brain.

The endocannabinoid system plays a very important role in the body and has a huge network of cannabinoid receptors spread throughout the body.

Interestingly, scientists found that the body makes its own chemicals called Endocannabinoids that produce a relaxing sensation.

The endocannabinoid system is perhaps the most important physiological system involved in establishing and maintaining human health.

These cannabinoids fit tightly into the body's anti-inflammatory, neuroprotective and anti-epileptic receptors.

The best way I can explain it is think of the endocannabinoid system literally as a bridge between our body and our mind.

And if the endocannabinoid system is out of balance, our whole body can be out of balance.

CBD activates cannabinoid receptors in the endocannabinoid system, like the adenosine and serotonin receptors.

Receptors are proteins that bind to ligands, which are ions and molecules, and cause responses in the immune system.

An example is the antigen receptor, which is involved in the release of dopamine and glutamate to neurotransmitters in the body.

CBD can boost these in adenosine levels in the brain. These specific receptors have anti-inflammatory effects throughout the body.

After reducing the inflammation, CBD is able to block pain signals from being sent to the brain.

CBD has been found to enhance serotonin receptors that influence symptoms of depression.

A research conducted in the University Of Sao Paulo, Brazil explored CBD and its effects on anxiety.

What they found is that high concentrations of CBD directly activates the serotonin receptor and causes an anti-anxiety effect.

The serotonin receptor is also involved in a number of neurological processes including addiction, appetite, and pain perception.

In 2013, the US National Library of Medicine published an experimental study which demonstrated that CBD could help with neurodegenerative disorders.

Neurodegenerative disorder is an umbrella term for a range of conditions which primarily affect the neurons in the human brain like Parkinson's disease.

CBD can also directly interact with the vanilloid receptors which function to mediate pain perception, inflammation and even body temperature.

In a particular human study, researchers used imaging scans to understand which brain regions are involved with CBDs anti-anxiety effects.

They found that CBD causes a reduction in blood flow to specific regions of the brain linked to anxiety such as hypothalamus.

The hypothalamus is a small area in the center of the brain that functions to regulate many essential functions in our body like appetite and weight control, emotions, sleep cycles, and sex drive.

These regions become overactive in anxiety disorders whereas CBD seems to quiet such activities.

CBD was also effective at reducing the overall anxiety of participants in the study.

CBD also boosts adenosine levels in the brain. These receptors have anti-inflammatory effects throughout the body.

CBD also works to manage pain by acting on the CB2 receptors which are mostly found in the peripheral nervous system.

By reducing inflammation, CBD is able to block pain signals from being sent to the brain.

Earlier, I mentioned the most prominent case of CBD being used to treat epilepsy in a girl named Charlotte who suffered from Dravet syndrome.

Dravet syndrome is a severe form of epilepsy in children and at one point caused Charlotte to suffer from over 300 seizures a week.

However after starting treatment with CBD rich oil, her seizures decreased dramatically to only two to three a month.

CBD appears to do this by lowering the degree of excitation of brain cells which contributes to seizures, and possibly migraines.

Another study found that the anti-psychotic effects of CBD are related to its effect on Anandamide.

Anandamide is a neurotransmitter produced in the brain that binds to the receptors.

It has been called the Bliss molecule and it's named after Ananda, the Sanskrit word for joy, bliss or happiness.

It is considered an endocannabinoid and it produces a state of heightened happiness and it is also important in memory motivation and for higher thought processes.

CBD has been found to increase levels of Anandamide in the brain which is linked to a decrease in psychotic symptoms.

The Journal of Neuroscience published a report back in 2013 that cannabinoids may help relieve migraines and help with neuropathic pain, such as nerve injury or other conditions which can predispose patients to developing nerve problems like diabetes or multiple sclerosis.

So the list goes on and on about the benefits of cannabidiol CBD on our bodies.

We are yet in the early stages of learning all the benefits of CBD. And what may work for some may not work for others.

Make sure you check with your doctor if you are suffering from a chronic disease or taking certain medications to ensure that CBD oil is safe for you to use.

Also remember not all CBD oil is created equal and as its popularity grows so will the demand.

You don't want to end up with inferior or unsafe CBD oil so please do your research.

ENDOCANNABINOID SYSTEM: HOW IT WORKS

When cannabinoids are introduced into the body, they will go the receptor sites and activate them.

And they will do all that is required to transform the system in your body in order to get the needed balance back into your body.

There are two different types of CB receptors in the body's endocannabinoid system.

The first one is found through a range of different areas in the brain.

And the second, which is more peripherally located, tends to be more related to the immune system.

However, when diseases occur, there tends to be an occurrence of these receptor sites wherever they're needed.

The purpose of the CB1 and CB2 receptor sites and the endocannabinoid system is to achieve homeostasis.

And when you have a homeostatic system, things work together the way they are supposed to.

The presence of disease implies a lack of homeostasis within the body.

Anandamide is this mediator of the central endocannabinoid system in the body and the interesting thing is that CBD has an indirect relationship to the amount of Anandamide in the system and that in turn triggers the endocannabinoid system.

Even though there is a big trend towards CBD only, and people are somehow freaked out about the side effects of psychoactivity- and euphoria and Happiness are listed as negative side effects of thc.

One thing that I cannot but mention is that without THC, you're leaving the vast majority of diagnoses and diseases and most sick people without treatment because THC has more mechanisms of action and medical application than you can imagine.

In fact frequently with epilepsy, where CBD maybe works for a while or stops working, THC might be what's needed in its place.

And in all those cases you still have to have a little bit of THC.

CBD of course is being studied as an antipsychotic, antiepileptic, improvement of extreme anti-inflammatory.

It's a wonderful tool for inflammation and pain management and also in keeping cancer cells from coming back.

CBD OIL TYPES FOR BEGINNERS

Getting to know the types of CBD oil out there will help know which is best for you so that you can make determined decisions when you shop for CBD oil.

Here, we will be looking at three types of CBD oil; the tincture drops, vape (pen and shot) and pure oil concentrates.

We will go into some brief details about each, such as their characteristics, potency, and how long lasting their effects are.

Tincture Drops

The tincture drops variant of CBD oil comes in the drop off bottles and diluted in carrier oils. You use it sublingually by dropping the liquid off the tip of its holder.

The liquid may either be flavored (tasty drops) or otherwise.

If you prefer to have something close to the raw cannabis plants itself and would want that to be in tincture drop form, the tasty drops might just fit your bill.

Tasty drops come raw and unheated. Which means it still has its CO_2 content, hence cannabidiol CBD-A, which is absent in other heated products.

CBD oil tincture drops lose their CO_2 content when heated. This increases its potency and effectiveness. With CBD-A transformed to just CBD by heating, the decarboxylated CBD oil is left with a stronger and higher in the concentration of CBD.

Vape

The two major categories of this are the vape shots and the refillable vape pens. The later has a disposable cartridge with relatively good CBD concentration.

About ninety percent of consumed vape CBD oil gets into the bloodstream so you are likely to get most out of what you consume.

And not just that, it also very potent and strong and gets into the system very fast, especially the vape shot which is easier to use and get going.

Vape shots or refill can be flavored with either natural plant-based or artificial flavors such as vegetable glycerin or propane glycol. The downside is that artificially flavored oils become toxic when heated.

Always remember, vape liquids are to be used in vape pens only. Don't be tempted to use it with tincture drops because the liquid will easily clot the tip.

And to cap it up, you may be required to vape several times daily, because the effects are usually short term.

Pure Oil Concentrates

As the name implies, pure oil comes with no oil carriers or added flavors. It is a pure extract of the hemp plant, has a more grassy taste, and has the greatest potency.

Pure oil concentrates also come in different forms; raw, blue label and gold label, with the raw form being closest to the raw hemp plant. The raw pure oil concentrate also has the CBD-A, which means it's still got its CO_2 content. Nothing added, nothing taken.

On the other hand, the blue label, which has been heated, has now become blue in color with a larger composition of CBD and greater potency.

The gold label is somewhat similar to the blue label, heated and potent.

But the residue plant components have been filtered off, leaving it with the greatest potency and highest concentration of CBD.

The gold label is most preferred, partly due to its potency and partly because it's not likely to mess up your mouth and teeth, unlike the blue label.

Pure oil concentrates last longer than the vape pens or shot. The best way to use the pure oil concentrate is sublingual that is, applied under your tongue.

It may also be added to food like honey and ingested but at the price of a lower absorption rate which normally should take any time around 20 minutes.

This is far from what you will be getting if added to food and you might as well not use it at all.

HOW MUCH CBD SHOULD I TAKE AS A BEGINNER?

There is a need to understand the difference between percentages of CBD, and milligrams of CBD. So that when you're going to buy a CBD product, you know exactly what you need to buy.

If you are starting out on your CBD journey, what is recommended is to take just 10 milligrams of CBD a day.

After 7 days of taking 10 milligrams a day, if you feel it necessary, you can double it and take 20 milligrams a day.

You could take 10 milligrams in the morning and 10 milligrams in the evening.

After another 7 days, if you feel it necessary, you can double it again.

Now, a maximum daily amount of CBD that is recommended here is 200 milligrams.

There have been clinical trials whereby they have tested 1500 milligrams on patients but those are simply trials and they were carried out by competent medical professionals.

But you should be fine with a maximum daily allowance of 200 milligrams.

Percentage of CBD versus Milligrams of CBD

A popular question that is being asked on a daily basis is how much CBD percentage is in the bottle.

Percentage of CBD is not a good way to choose a CBD product.

For example, you may think that 25% CBD oil has got more CBD in it than the 15% CBD oil.

However, the 25% CBD may only have 250 milligrams of CBD whereas the 15% may have up to 450 milligrams of the CBD Concentrate.

It is really important to know how much milligrams you are getting per serving when you're buying a CBD product.

Companies that are members of the cannabis and hemp associations in the United States will follow guidelines for their labeling so it will be really easy for you to understand how many milligrams of the CBD you are getting per serving.

However, not all companies in the United States and abroad will follow these same guidelines for labeling.

Some labels could be a bit confusing, even though the product may be fantastic; you literally have to work out the milligrams per serving, by having to divide the total amount of CBD by the number of servings.

So for every 'N' drops of CBD oil, you get 'X' milligrams of CBD.

Now that example of a label is very confusing and it may take quite some time to work it out.

So you want to be mindful of the labeling whenever you are out to buy CBD oil.

HOW LONG DO CBD OIL EFFECTS LAST?

In terms of the half-life for cannabidiol, the range is somewhere between 21 hours and 48 hours. So it's a fairly long half-life.

People also talk about an inverted u-shaped dose curve.

What that means is that you don't see much effect at low doses, and then you see a significant effect at moderate doses, and then the effect seems to fall off.

The question of how long the effect of CBD Oil itself lasts is quite popular and it is a really good question.

It also matters so much because when you are buying your CBD oil, you want to get something that is not only going to work, but also work for a longer period so that you are not going to have to reuse too frequently.

How long CBD will act after consumption varies from person to person.

It can vary from 1 hour for one person taking a product to 12 hours for another person taking the same exact product.

So here, I intend to give you general guidelines to help equip you when you do buy your CBD oil.

The different types are going to generally last different lengths of time, so let's start with the vaping.

Vaping

The vaping CBD is an electric cigarette pen that you put the vaping liquid in.

Remember; do not put the tincture drops in your vape pen because it will clog it up.

The vape liquid has a high efficacy of about 90%, which means that it is going to get into your bloodstream fast, typically within five minutes.

However its effect is usually short, typically anywhere from two to three hours is a general idea of how long the CBD will last with vaping.

Therefore, you will have to vape more often. Next is the tincture drops.

The Tincture Drops

The tincture drops can last about 4 to 5 hours.

This also depends on the person. Its efficacy is going to be a little bit lower than both the vape and the pure oil concentrates.

This simply means you are not going to absorb much of the CBD. The effects are going to last approximately four to five hours.

The Pure Oil Concentrates

The pure oil concentrates which could either be paste or gel comes in a syringe tube.

Those are going to have a bit higher efficacy than the tincture drops, typically up to 75% efficacy.

So you get a lot out of it and it absorbs better into the system when you sublingually hold it under your tongue.

The effects are going to last anywhere from 5 to 12 hours.

Some people only need to take the pure oil concentrate once. If you have a high level of pain, you might have to take it two or three times a day.

But it's quite rare for anyone having to take it more than three times a day.

What you could do with the pure oil concentrate is to start with once a day and see how long it lasts, then maybe bump it up to two times a day if you need to.

That is how you want to try all of these different types.

You want to start with the recommended dosing instead of starting with a bigger quantity unless you're using it for insomnia, in which case you can use a bigger quantity before you go to bed.

But you might want to see how the amount that you use works first and then try a little bit more to kind of get the amount and the length of time that it's going to last.

So start with once a day and wait half an hour. If you don't feel any effects, go ahead take a little bit more and wait another half an hour and see if that worked for you.

That's how you find your dosage and then the type that you are going to choose is going to be based on whether you need immediate results, in which case, vaping would be preferred. But you won't mind having to do that several times a day.

If you want something that's going to have a longer lasting effect, you should go for the pure oil concentrates.

And then the tincture drops is going to fall somewhere in the middle.

There are also capsules and edibles available for purchase but if you are really sick and you are having a weak digestive system, capsules and edibles don't work.

In order to take capsules and edibles, you need to have a good digestive system to even digest and absorb the CBD.

Also, the efficacy is going to be very low when it has to go through the entire digestive system

.

IS CBD OIL LEGAL?

Not only is Google confused, but lawmakers are confused as well, the public is also confused about whether it is legal, chiefly because they can't even define exactly what it is.

Hemp is legal in all 50 states according to the 2014 farm bill.

Marijuana is legal in some states for medicinal and/or recreational purposes.

Some states permit the recreational use of cannabis, other states say it's illegal, but in all 50 states, CBD products that are extracted from hemp are legal.

It is also very interesting to know that the United States Federal Government owns the patent on cannabinoids.

CBD oil is not quite a legal product world over. While hemp base CBD is legal in most places, CBD oil is not legal in every country, especially if it's derived from high THC cannabis plants.

Please check your local laws to find out the legality in your country.

Is It Safe For You To Take CBD Oil?

CBD is absolutely harmless.

It is completely natural and according to physicians, there are no side effects and there are no contradictions.

You don't have to worry about the possibility of taking it with some medications.

It is also important to find a holistic practitioner that believes in the healing properties of CBD oil. It's always good to integrate them into your care.

It is quite obvious that western medical practitioners that haven't embraced it, don't understand it, and turn it away.

That is because they are not educated about it, and it's not within their realm of practice.

It's actually is a natural human behavior to turn something away that you're not really familiar with.

But I can tell you, the holistic community, for example, the acupuncturist or anybody in the holistic and wellness space, have totally embraced it.

They don't even need to be told what it is anymore.

They already know about it and have seen the benefits. So it is completely safe.

But again if you consult a practitioner about it, make sure you're asking a practitioner who is open and educated about what CBD is.

Does CBD Have Any Side Effects?

CBD has been proven to have very few side effects.

In some studies, a small group of people experienced effects like lightheadedness, drowsiness, dry mouth, and diarrhea.

Probably, what's most important to know is that CBD can inhibit hepatic drug metabolism in few cases.

So if you are using medication, it is best to check with your doctor to make sure that CBD is not going to have any effect on the medication you are taking

Can You Fail A Drug Test Taking CBD Oil?

In the field of medicine, drug tests are carried out on patients for a number of reasons.

Sometimes it's because what interacts with whatever is in the system, and the cause of some symptoms needs to be known.

For example, you may have a patient that goes to the hospital with a chest pain, it can easily be assumed to be a heart attack or something related. But when the drug screen is pulled, it may show that there is a lot of cocaine in the system.

So, the drug screens are used determine what's in the system and how to approach it.

CBD oil is still a new product in the marketplace and one of the things that people are concerned about is if they can get high or fail a drug test in the course of using it.

There are people that work for the law enforcement, people that work in schools, and the military. These people are genuinely concerned.

Since there is no THC, is it less likely that you will fail drug test using CBD oil because it only has the nonpsychoactive CBD and all of these other cannabinoids in it.

There is just such a minuscule trace amount of THC, so it's safe to say that there is negligible THC in CBD oils.

Drug screening is actually looking for THC and not cannabis because if that were the case, it means anything you take with hemp in it, would pop positive on a drug screen. CBD oil will not produce a positive result on the drug screen.

A urine drug screen is a ten-panel drug screen. It is looking for ten different things; methamphetamine, opioid, cocaine, THC and so on. If you ate poppy seed bagel every single day, that doesn't mean you are doing cocaine.

What the actual drug test looking for in THC is an actual number, a threshold.

Usually, it's like thirty milligrams of THC in your system. So for that, you'd have to actually be smoking marijuana within 72 hours to test positive.

If you have any concerns, it's really easy to go to Amazon to order a urine drug test and test your own urine. You can get maybe 10 of them for seven dollars.

So if that concern is there, you should definitely do it yourself. The urine test works just like a pregnancy test.

It gives you your result within two minutes in your bathroom and on top of that, it's going to basically produce the same results that you would get whenever you go in for your employment drug screen.

PART 2: HOW TO BUY CBD OIL PROPER

INTRODUCTION

The markets for CBD oil is rising and will continue to rise as long as science and reviews continue to endorse it.

CBD oil is available for purchase online and at physical health and food stores across the country.

However, the quality of CBD oil depends largely on factors such as methods of extraction, storage, and packaging processes.

Unfortunately, due to lack of expertise in rightly managing these factors, the market today is flooded with as many low-quality products (if not more) as quality CBD oils.

So you need to be careful in making your purchases so that you can always get the results you desire.

The plant, cannabis sativa can be subdivided into two categories; hemp or cannabis.

It all boils down to the amount of THC.

According to the Section 7606 of the Agricultural Act of 2014; hemp is defined as having less than 0.3 percent THC and therefore by default, cannabis has more than 0.3 percent THC.

So hemp and cannabis come from the same plant species and the distinction between the two is a legal one.

Basically, hemp CBD oil has less THC in it and cannabis CBD oil has more THC.

Whether there is an advantage or even a disadvantage to having more or less THC entirely depends on the medical condition that you're treating.

The general perception out there is that CBD has all the medical value when it comes to either hemp or marijuana.

But in fact, that's not the case.

Some medical conditions benefit from more CBD and others from more THC, and then there are some medical conditions that benefit from both THC and CBD.

So if you have a condition that doesn't benefit from the use of CBD, then it's not an option worth pursuing, it's a waste of your money.

In terms of chemical structure, the CBD and hemp are the same as the CBD in cannabis.

It's coming from the same plant and your body is going to recognize the CBD in hemp the same way as CBD in cannabis.

WHERE TO BUY

There are a couple different places that people buy cannabis and/or hemp CBD oil from.

Medical Marijuana Dispensary

One is at a medical marijuana dispensary in a state where marijuana has been deemed legal for either medical or recreational use.

Some of these states have regulations in place to assure the quality of the products being sold at these medical marijuana dispensaries.

Online

People purchase hemp CBD oil through websites on the internet but as it stands, there are no regulations in place to assure the quality of the products being sold through websites on the Internet.

In 2015 and in 2016, the FDA, otherwise known as the Food and Drug Administration, ran some tests on CBD products sold through these websites on the Internet.

In some of these products, CBD wasn't detected at all or it paled in comparison to the claim that was made on the label.

For example, one product label which claimed 50 milligrams of CBD actually tested negative for cannabinoids.

Another claim made on the label said 21% CBD, but it tested negative for cannabinoids

Now in another example where the claim made on the label said 26% CBD, they only detected 0.14 percent CBD.

To make matters worse, some of these products actually had more than 0.3% THC in them.

Now of course for obvious reasons the FDA sent out warning letters to these companies because they were making untruthful claims about the amount of CBD in their products.

And also some companies were selling products that actually had more than federally legal amounts of THC in them.

HOW TO BUY

It's no wonder that some patients report that they purchased supposed hemp CBD oil product through a website on the internet and either it didn't work.

Or they actually felt high off of the product that they purchased.

For this reason, I've come up with a list of questions for patients to ask sellers when buying CBD oil.

As the industry stays unregulated, you are bound to find salesmen that will make all sorts of unqualified claims about their products to make a quick buck.

So really it's on you to be a smart consumer.

Purchasing CBD Oil: What To Look Out For.

Below is a list of criteria you should use when buying CBD oil.

Sourcing

Is it domestically grown and manufactured?

There's a tremendous confusion about the quality of CBD, and looking at the CBD landscape, the vast majority of products that's out there is not from whole plants.

So, there is a need for you to be educated about what the difference is and how do they know when you are looking for CBD products.

From an herbalist standpoint, whole plant extracts are extremely important.

The Entourage Effect

Botanical medicine has been around for thousands of years in our evolution.

And whenever you extract a plant, you get all of those other molecules, hundreds or sometimes thousands of molecules, and they work in a beautiful mix together in the body.

The body understands that because we have been evolving with these plants.

We have been eating them.

We have been using them as medicine for thousands of years.

Our bodies can recognize all of those other secondary molecules in there

They can act to help balance out these materials in our body.

A lot of times it's called the Entourage Effect or Synergy.

This is just the natural way we have been healing ourselves for thousands of years.

So when the single compounds are pulled away from all of those other secondary molecules, your balance can completely go out of whack because it doesn't have those other balancing methods within it.

You can get serious side effects like we see from a lot of synthesized pharmaceuticals.

As a consumer, you need to look into the manufacturer and check to see where they are sourcing material.

This is because these minor cannabinoids or other molecules that are just being discovered, and the ones that we have discovered like terpenes, flavonoids all work together to bring out the best benefit out of CBD Oil.

A lot of hemp is still coming from overseas like China and Europe and there is no way for us to know the genetics, how it is grown, and how it's being monitored.

These factors determine its consistency and potency.

You should also know that the hemp plant is a bio-accumulator.

Where it's grown matters a lot because it can accumulate toxins, heavy metals, and things like that.

If the plant is grown on a toxic land, it becomes toxic.

So where the plant is grown is extremely important.

Are the varieties and genetics the same?

Is it going to be consistent?

Is it a whole plant extract?

These things are very important.

As the consumer, you need to know the process and the folks who are supplying these products should be able to show the process, show the efficacy, and show certificates of analysis and testing.

Accountability

Is the maker of the CBD oil accountable to anyone?

Is the company trustworthy?

It's when a company is not accountable that they may use deceptive and misleading marketing and advertising, and get away with it.

Now in some states where marijuana is legal for either medical or recreational use, there are rules and regulations in place that the makers of the CBD oils have to abide by.

So for patients in these states where marijuana is legal for medical and or recreational use, you are better off purchasing the CBD oil from state-licensed facilities that are authorized to specifically dispense marijuana and hemp products.

Laboratory Tested

Is the product laboratory tested?

Has it been tested by third-party?

The company that made the product should be able to present to you the most recent laboratory test results for the product.

And at the very least; the laboratory test results should indicate the exact amounts of THC and CBD in the product.

Is it Full-Spectrum or Isolate?

What Is Full-Spectrum CBD Oil?

Full-spectrum CBD oil includes all 80 plus cannabinoids; terpenes, flavonoids and other molecules that are beneficial in the hemp plant.

Having all of these cannabinoids working together synergistically creates what is known as the Entourage Effect.

That is when you get the medicinal benefits that everybody's talking about.

There is also what's called CBD Isolate which is the opposite of full-spectrum CBD, and it is exactly as the name sounds: CBD isolated from the oil.

It does not contain any other cannabinoids from the hemp plant.

It looks like a fine white powder.

It is not synthetic or lab made.

It is an all-natural product

It normally has a purity level of about 99%, and

It is the most potent CBD product available if you are just looking for CBD.

It can be added to oil or sold as CBD only.

Extraction

In addition to the full spectrum, it is important to have the oil extracted from the whole plant.

That means the leaves, the flowers, and the stalks; these are the most valuable parts of the plant.

Foreign hemp oil is extracted from the stalks only.

Though imported hemp extracted just from the stalks used to be legal, it's no longer the case.

There are several companies out there that are still stating that that's the only way to legally consume oil in the United States, but that is simply not correct.

Means of Extraction

Many times CBD is extracted in a hydrocarbon like butane which can be harmful to your health.

So check to ask what the CBD was extracted in.

Cannabinoids cannot be extracted from hemp seeds as some websites claim.

There are no cannabinoids that originate from the seed.

The seed has great omega fatty acids which are important.

It is better to use hemp seed oil as the carrier oil because the cannabinoids are actually absorbed into our system better when you have fatty oil.

If a website says THC or CBD is being extracted from the seed, it's false.

There may be trace elements just because it comes from the same plant, but it is not a source.

Methods of Extraction

The extraction process is also important.

CO2 Extraction

The most technologically advanced method is the CO2 Extraction.

This requires more skill and a greater cost, which automatically is going to eliminate some companies from the marketplace.

It uses carbon dioxide under high pressure and low temperatures, to isolate, preserve and maintain the purity of the oil.

This method allows an extractor to separate the cannabinoids and ultimately introduce only those that are desired.

This is a better way to remove the THC.

It's very safe, potent and free of any chlorophyll.

Alcohol Extraction

Alcohol Extraction is another method of extraction that is fairly popular.

The plant is soaked in high-grade alcohol and then when it evaporates, you're left with the oil.

Although I described how to extract your own homemade cannabis CBD oil later in this book, this extraction method destroys the plant waxes which may have health benefits.

Olive Oil Extraction

In addition to that, there are olive oil methods of extraction.

This is something that is used by many companies.

It is considered safe and inexpensive.

However, it is perishable and should be stored in a cool dark place.

The downside with this method is it reduces the CBD concentration.

So you would have to consume large quantities to receive any medicinal benefits.

Third Party Testing

Another thing that is very important is you want oils that are third-party tested.

This is critical because you want to make sure that there are no toxins in the oil you are consuming.

You also want to be sure that that your CBD oil is pure and potent.

So when you're shopping, make sure that you ask for the third-party testing results so that you can be sure that you are getting a quality product.

This plays very well with company transparency.

If the company is not willing to share that information, then you should consider using another vendor.

So make sure before you buy, you can answer those questions or you are going to buy a product that may not give you the results.

And then you may be misled to believe that perhaps the product does not work when in actuality, CBD oil does work when it is full spectrum.

You might have bought an isolate and thought that it was going to take away your pain.

There are quality products out there.

But you have to be able to answer the questions to make sure that you are getting your money's worth.

CBD OIL APPLICATION: A PRACTICAL GUIDE FOR BEGINNERS

As a beginner, a good place to start is right at the packaging.

Reference Point

The recommended dosing is basic.

You need to get familiar with the suggested servings indicated on the package.

Read the instructions carefully.

As you begin to use it, the results you see and/or reactions will determine how much to add or how much reduction is needed for desired results.

So, the recommended serving is always the reference point.

Results

Expectations and results largely depend on which type of the oil you are going to be using; pure, vape or tincture drops.

The different types tend to kick in into the system at different times after use and depending on the method of use.

The onset time for vape is typically 5 to 10 minutes.

If added to food, pure oil concentrates may take as long as an hour to fully absorb into the system.

Otherwise, the onset time may vary between 20 to 45 minutes when used orally.

The drops are harder to hold sublingually and the onset time should last between 30 to 45 minutes.

It is no surprise that an average first time user normally expects immediate results from this drug.

Sometimes that happens; however, it may take about a week for the full effects of CBD to kick in especially for pain related issues.

Meaning that CBD oil does work wonders, but not instantaneously every time.

Some users have reported experiencing a feeling of calmness and/or a reduction in racing thoughts after first use.

This happens a lot.

Inflammations may also reduce quickly after the first serving.

Those suffering from anxiety and sleep-related issues tend to experience fastest results.

Some users go to sleep not long after the first serving.

However, full sleep cycle regularization can also take some time to reach a significant level.

So whether or not you feel the effects of CBD oil use instantly, CBD oil is an amazing drug and you will see tangible results in little time.

Also, as with most nutritious foods or drugs when ingested, after your couple of first servings, you may start to experience symptoms that arise from detoxification, such as brief dizziness, fatigue, slight headaches, or even skin breaks.

This happens because when nutritious foods enter into the system they push out toxic wastes into the bloodstream.

So it's not a side effect per say.

When you experience these symptoms, you can flush the toxins out of the bloodstream by drinking lots of water, and participating in deep breathing exercises.

If the symptoms persist after a few days, reduce the frequency of use.

If you have been taking the oil once every day, you may switch to once every two days.

Do this and observe the difference.

Reset

You may also need to give your body some time to recover. You can do this by stopping your use of the oil for a little while.

We all have different body makeup. You have to understand that this can even happen at first encounter with any other drug or food.

In all, you need to exercise needed patience if you must reap the immense benefits of CBD oil.

Not that it's weird to expect tangible results overnight, but it doesn't always happen that way.

9 STEPS TO MAKE YOUR OWN HOME MADE CBD OIL

I have chosen to add this for information purposes only.

In order to make CBD oil at home you need;

- A lighter
- Coffee machine
- Sieve
- Pure alcohol
- Small bowls
- Big bowl
- Cannabis (Good plant material: in order to make a nice extract)
- Coffee filters

I will show you how to extract CBD oil from cannabis using *Ethanol*.

It is extremely important you use the organic material so that you know there is nothing inside that can harm you.

It is equally important that you choose a variety of cannabis plant that has a high concentration of CBD.

There are over 4,000 different varieties of the cannabis plant.

Follow these simple steps to make your own CBD oil at home:

Step 1

Take a bowl and put the plant material inside.

Step 2

Pour enough ethanol to cover the plant material.

The usefulness of the ethanol is to separate the plant material from the cannabinoids.

You need to be very fast with this process because you don't want the ethanol to be in contact with the plant material for a long time.

If that happens, you get a lot of other stuff inside which you don't want.

Step 3

Use a plastic spoon to stir for about three minutes.

Do not use mechanical mixers to avoid creating a spark.

If by any chance a spark is created, everything will burn.

Step 4

After mixing, separate the ethanol from the plant material using a sieve and another bowl.

This is the first filtration.

Now you are going to do the second filtration in order to remove the plant material you have left.

This is where you use the coffee machine.

The machine can heat your material and it can filter.

Start with the filtration part.

Step 5

Scoop the material with your spoon through the coffee filter paper into the coffee machine.

In order to accelerate the process, you can change the paper every time a single filtration has occurred.

If the plant material is much, you need to continue until it does not contain any more plant material.

Step 7

Now it is time to separate the ethanol from the cannabinoids.

You can either cook to vaporize the ethanol or use a water distiller instead.

The water distiller is my favorite because you will have to cook outdoors in the open air.

But to make it all easier, use the water distiller.

The time required for full separation depends on how much material you put inside.

Use a bowl to collect the pure ethanol that's going to come out because you can reuse it again and again.

Switch it on and wait.

When you have up to 80% of the original ethanol volume, open the lid slowly and look inside to check what's going on, stop when you see very little material left in the distiller.

Stand back for a few moments to avoid breathing it in.

And be careful when you pour so that you don't lose the little extract you have.

Step 8

Use the coffee machine to remove the remaining ethanol from your extract.

Put it on the heating device, turn it on and wait for 24 hours at least so that you're sure that no ethanol is left.

Don't be surprised if you have very little oil after all the effort.

Step 9

The final test is a quality test.

Dip a paper clip into the material and light it to see what happens.

If there is a spark you know there is ethanol left in the mixture, in that case, you need to put it back on the heater.

Keep heating until you don't get any sparks anymore.

Enjoy your cannabis extract.

CONCLUSION

CBD is a fantastic plant and misconceptions need to be eliminated. This is an industry that is growing. In fact, it is estimated to be a 2.1 billion dollar industry by 2020. That means there is going to be a lot of players entering the marketplace.

But, unfortunately, there is not a lot of regulation, so it is your responsibility as a consumer to know what you're buying so you get the desired results.

While it may be practically impossible to meet everyone's every need,

I do hope you gained relevant information from this book. Your reviews are highly welcome. Thank you.

44641389R00064

Made in the USA
Middletown, DE
08 May 2019